Exercise Log Book
Fitness & Strength Tracking Progress

Daily Workout Log   Date:_____________

Pre-Exercise Meal / Snack:_________________________

Energy Level Before Workout: L   M   H

Weight:__________   Sleep:__________   Calories:__________

Cardio

Type:____

Time:______________   Distance:________________

Heart Rate:________________   Intensity: L   M   H

Strength Training

Exercise	Sets	Reps	Wt	Rest

Notes / Comments

____

____

____

Daily Workout Log   Date: _____________

Pre-Exercise Meal / Snack: ______________________________

Energy Level Before Workout: L   M   H

Weight: _________   Sleep: _________   Calories: _________

Cardio

Type: ____

Time: _______________   Distance: _______________

Heart Rate: _______________   Intensity: L   M   H

Strength Training

Exercise	Sets	Reps	Wt	Rest

Notes / Comments

____

____

____

Daily Workout Log   Date: __________

Pre-Exercise Meal / Snack: _____________________

Energy Level Before Workout: L   M   H

Weight: ________   Sleep: _________   Calories: ________

Cardio

Type: ___________________________________

Time: ____________   Distance: _____________

Heart Rate: _____________   Intensity: L   M   H

Strength Training

Exercise	Sets	Reps	Wt	Rest

Notes / Comments

____

____

____

Daily Workout Log

Date: _________

Pre-Exercise Meal / Snack: _____________________

Energy Level Before Workout: L   M   H

Weight: _______   Sleep: ________   Calories: _______

Cardio

Type: ____

Time: ____________   Distance: ____________

Heart Rate: _____________   Intensity: L   M   H

Strength Training

Exercise	Sets	Reps	Wt	Rest

Notes / Comments

____

____

____

Daily Workout Log Date: ___________

Pre-Exercise Meal / Snack: _____________________

Energy Level Before Workout: L   M   H

Weight: _________   Sleep: _________   Calories: _________

Cardio

Type: _______________________________________

Time: _____________   Distance: _______________

Heart Rate: _______________   Intensity: L   M   H

Strength Training

Exercise	Sets	Reps	Wt	Rest

Notes / Comments

____

____

____

Daily Workout Log   Date: __________

Pre-Exercise Meal / Snack: ____________________

Energy Level Before Workout: L   M   H

Weight: _________   Sleep: _________   Calories: ________

Cardio

Type: _______________________________________

Time: ____________   Distance: ______________

Heart Rate: ______________   Intensity: L   M   H

Strength Training

Exercise	Sets	Reps	Wt	Rest

Notes / Comments

____

____

____

Daily Workout Log　　Date: _________

Pre-Exercise Meal / Snack: ____________________

Energy Level Before Workout:　L　　M　　H

Weight: ________　　Sleep: ________　　Calories: ________

Cardio

Type: _____________________________________

Time: ____________　　　　Distance: ______________

Heart Rate: _____________　　Intensity: L　　M　　H

Strength Training

Exercise	Sets	Reps	Wt	Rest

Notes / Comments

____

____

____

Daily Workout Log

Date: ___________

Pre-Exercise Meal / Snack: _____________________

Energy Level Before Workout: L   M   H

Weight: _________   Sleep: _________   Calories: _________

Cardio

Type: ____

Time: _____________   Distance: _______________

Heart Rate: _______________   Intensity: L   M   H

Strength Training

Exercise	Sets	Reps	Wt	Rest

Notes / Comments

____

____

____

Daily Workout Log   Date: _________

Pre-Exercise Meal / Snack: ____________________

Energy Level Before Workout: L   M   H

Weight: _______   Sleep: ________   Calories: _______

Cardio

Type: _________________________________

Time: ___________   Distance: _____________

Heart Rate: _____________   Intensity: L   M   H

Strength Training

Exercise	Sets	Reps	Wt	Rest

Notes / Comments

____

____

____

Daily Workout Log   Date: __________

Pre-Exercise Meal / Snack: ____________________

Energy Level Before Workout: L   M   H

Weight: ________   Sleep: ________   Calories: _______

Cardio

Type: ____

Time: ___________   Distance: ____________

Heart Rate: _____________   Intensity: L   M   H

Strength Training

Exercise	Sets	Reps	Wt	Rest

Notes / Comments

____

____

____

Daily Workout Log   Date: _____________

Pre-Exercise Meal / Snack: ____________________________

Energy Level Before Workout: L   M   H

Weight: _________   Sleep: _________   Calories: _________

Cardio

Type: ____

Time: _______________   Distance: _______________

Heart Rate: _______________   Intensity: L   M   H

Strength Training

Exercise	Sets	Reps	Wt	Rest

Notes / Comments

____

____

____

Daily Workout Log   Date: _____________

Pre-Exercise Meal / Snack: _________________________

Energy Level Before Workout: L   M   H

Weight: _________   Sleep: _________   Calories: _________

Cardio

Type: ____

Time: _____________   Distance: _______________

Heart Rate: _______________   Intensity: L   M   H

Strength Training

Exercise	Sets	Reps	Wt	Rest

Notes / Comments

____

____

____

Daily Workout Log   Date: _____________

Pre-Exercise Meal / Snack: _______________________________

Energy Level Before Workout: L   M   H

Weight: _________   **Sleep:** _________   **Calories:** _________

Cardio

Type: ____

Time: _____________   **Distance:** _______________

Heart Rate: ________________   **Intensity:** L   M   H

Strength Training

Exercise	Sets	Reps	Wt	Rest

Notes / Comments

____

____

____

Daily Workout Log   Date: __________

Pre-Exercise Meal / Snack: ___________________

Energy Level Before Workout: L   M   H

Weight: _______   Sleep: _______   Calories: _______

Cardio

Type: ___________________________________

Time: ___________   Distance: ___________

Heart Rate: ___________   Intensity: L   M   H

Strength Training

Exercise	Sets	Reps	Wt	Rest

Notes / Comments

____

____

____

Daily Workout Log

Date: _____________

Pre-Exercise Meal / Snack: _______________________

Energy Level Before Workout: L   M   H

Weight: __________   Sleep: __________   Calories: __________

Cardio

Type: _______________________________________

Time: _______________   Distance: ________________

Heart Rate: _______________   Intensity: L   M   H

Strength Training

Exercise	Sets	Reps	Wt	Rest

Notes / Comments

____

____

____

Daily Workout Log

Date: ___________

Pre-Exercise Meal / Snack: ____________________

Energy Level Before Workout: L   M   H

Weight: _______   Sleep: ________   Calories: _______

Cardio

Type: ________________________________

Time: ____________   Distance: ______________

Heart Rate: ______________   Intensity: L   M   H

Strength Training

Exercise	Sets	Reps	Wt	Rest

Notes / Comments

____

____

____

Daily Workout Log   Date: __________

Pre-Exercise Meal / Snack: _______________________

Energy Level Before Workout: L   M   H

Weight: ________   Sleep: ________   Calories: ________

Cardio

Type: ____

Time: ____________   Distance: _______________

Heart Rate: _______________   Intensity: L   M   H

Strength Training

Exercise	Sets	Reps	Wt	Rest

Notes / Comments

____

____

____

Daily Workout Log   Date:__________

Pre-Exercise Meal / Snack:___________________

Energy Level Before Workout: L   M   H

Weight:_________   Sleep:_________   Calories:________

Cardio

Type:____

Time:____________   Distance:______________

Heart Rate:_____________   Intensity: L   M   H

Strength Training

Exercise	Sets	Reps	Wt	Rest

Notes / Comments

____

____

____

Daily Workout Log

Date: _____________

Pre-Exercise Meal / Snack: _____________________

Energy Level Before Workout: L   M   H

Weight: _________   Sleep: _________   Calories: _________

Cardio

Type: ____

Time: _____________   Distance: _____________

Heart Rate: _______________   Intensity: L   M   H

Strength Training

Exercise	Sets	Reps	Wt	Rest

Notes / Comments

____

____

____

Daily Workout Log

Date: ___________

Pre-Exercise Meal / Snack: _____________________

Energy Level Before Workout: L   M   H

Weight: _________   Sleep: _________   Calories: _________

Cardio

Type: _________________________________

Time: _____________   Distance: _______________

Heart Rate: _______________   Intensity: L   M   H

Strength Training

Exercise	Sets	Reps	Wt	Rest

Notes / Comments

____

____

____

Daily Workout Log   Date: _____________

Pre-Exercise Meal / Snack: _______________________

Energy Level Before Workout: L   M   H

Weight: _________   **Sleep:** _________   **Calories:** _________

Cardio

Type: ____

Time: _____________   **Distance:** _______________

Heart Rate: _______________   **Intensity:** L   M   H

Strength Training

Exercise	Sets	Reps	Wt	Rest

Notes / Comments

____

____

____

Daily Workout Log   Date: ___________

Pre-Exercise Meal / Snack: _______________________

Energy Level Before Workout: L   M   H

Weight: _________   Sleep: _________   Calories: _______

Cardio

Type: ____

Time: _____________   Distance: _____________

Heart Rate: _______________   Intensity: L   M   H

Strength Training

Exercise	Sets	Reps	Wt	Rest

Notes / Comments

____

____

____

Daily Workout Log

Date: __________

Pre-Exercise Meal / Snack: ____________________

Energy Level Before Workout: L   M   H

Weight: ________   Sleep: ________   Calories: ________

Cardio

Type: _________________________________

Time: ____________   Distance: ____________

Heart Rate: ____________   Intensity: L   M   H

Strength Training

Exercise	Sets	Reps	Wt	Rest

Notes / Comments

____

____

____

Daily Workout Log   Date: _________

Pre-Exercise Meal / Snack: ___________________

Energy Level Before Workout: L   M   H

Weight: _________   Sleep: _________   Calories: _________

Cardio

Type: ____

Time: _____________   Distance: _______________

Heart Rate: _______________   Intensity: L   M   H

Strength Training

Exercise	Sets	Reps	Wt	Rest

Notes / Comments

____

____

____

Daily Workout Log

Date: _____________

Pre-Exercise Meal / Snack: _______________________

Energy Level Before Workout: L   M   H

Weight: _________   Sleep: _________   Calories: _________

Cardio

Type: ____

Time: _____________   Distance: _______________

Heart Rate: _______________   Intensity: L   M   H

Strength Training

Exercise	Sets	Reps	Wt	Rest

Notes / Comments

____

____

____

Daily Workout Log

Date: ___________

Pre-Exercise Meal / Snack: ________________________

Energy Level Before Workout: L   M   H

Weight: _________   Sleep: _________   Calories: _______

Cardio

Type: ____

Time: ____________   Distance: _____________

Heart Rate: ______________   Intensity: L   M   H

Strength Training

Exercise	Sets	Reps	Wt	Rest

Notes / Comments

____

____

____

Daily Workout Log

Date: _________

Pre-Exercise Meal / Snack: _____________________

Energy Level Before Workout: L   M   H

Weight: _________   Sleep: _________   Calories: _________

Cardio

Type: _____________________________________

Time: _____________   Distance: ______________

Heart Rate: _______________   Intensity: L   M   H

Strength Training

Exercise	Sets	Reps	Wt	Rest

Notes / Comments

____

____

____

Daily Workout Log   Date: _____________

Pre-Exercise Meal / Snack: _______________________

Energy Level Before Workout: L   M   H

Weight: _________   Sleep: _________   Calories: _________

Cardio

Type: ____

Time: _______________   Distance: _______________

Heart Rate: _______________   Intensity: L   M   H

Strength Training

Exercise	Sets	Reps	Wt	Rest

Notes / Comments

____

____

____

Daily Workout Log

Date: __________

Pre-Exercise Meal / Snack: _____________________

Energy Level Before Workout: L   M   H

Weight: _________   Sleep: _________   Calories: _________

Cardio

Type: _______________________________________

Time: ____________   Distance: ______________

Heart Rate: ____________   Intensity: L   M   H

Strength Training

Exercise	Sets	Reps	Wt	Rest

Notes / Comments

____

____

____

Daily Workout Log

Date: ___________

Pre-Exercise Meal / Snack: ____________________________

Energy Level Before Workout: L   M   H

Weight: _________   Sleep: _________   Calories: ________

Cardio

Type: ____

Time: ____________   Distance: ______________

Heart Rate: _____________   Intensity: L   M   H

Strength Training

Exercise	Sets	Reps	Wt	Rest

Notes / Comments

____

____

____

Day 30 Notes On Fitness Progress

Action Plan

Daily Workout Log   Date: __________

Pre-Exercise Meal / Snack: ____________________

Energy Level Before Workout: L   M   H

Weight: ________   Sleep: ________   Calories: _______

Cardio

Type: ______________________________________

Time: ____________   Distance: _____________

Heart Rate: ____________   Intensity: L   M   H

Strength Training

Exercise	Sets	Reps	Wt	Rest

Notes / Comments

____

____

____

Daily Workout Log

Date: _____________

Pre-Exercise Meal / Snack: _____________________

Energy Level Before Workout: L   M   H

Weight: _________   Sleep: _________   Calories: _________

Cardio

Type: _____________________________________

Time: _____________   Distance: _______________

Heart Rate: _______________   Intensity: L   M   H

Strength Training

Exercise	Sets	Reps	Wt	Rest

Notes / Comments

____

____

____

Daily Workout Log

Date: _______________

Pre-Exercise Meal / Snack: _______________________

Energy Level Before Workout: L   M   H

Weight: _________   Sleep: _________   Calories: _________

Cardio

Type: _______________________________

Time: _______________   Distance: _______________

Heart Rate: _______________   Intensity: L   M   H

Strength Training

Exercise	Sets	Reps	Wt	Rest

Notes / Comments

____

____

____

Daily Workout Log

Date:_____________

Pre-Exercise Meal / Snack:_____________________

Energy Level Before Workout: L   M   H

Weight:_________   Sleep:_________   Calories:_________

Cardio

Type:_______________________________________

Time:_____________   Distance:_______________

Heart Rate:_______________   Intensity: L   M   H

Strength Training

Exercise	Sets	Reps	Wt	Rest

Notes / Comments

____

____

____

Daily Workout Log   Date: _____________

Pre-Exercise Meal / Snack: _______________________

Energy Level Before Workout: L   M   H

Weight: _________   **Sleep:** _________   **Calories:** _________

Cardio

Type: ____

Time: _____________   **Distance:** _______________

Heart Rate: _______________   **Intensity:** L   M   H

Strength Training

Exercise	Sets	Reps	Wt	Rest

Notes / Comments

____

____

____

Daily Workout Log   Date:_________

Pre-Exercise Meal / Snack: _____________________

Energy Level Before Workout: L   M   H

Weight:________   Sleep:________   Calories:_______

Cardio

Type:____

Time:____________   Distance:_____________

Heart Rate:____________   Intensity: L   M   H

Strength Training

Exercise	Sets	Reps	Wt	Rest

Notes / Comments

____

____

____

Daily Workout Log   Date:_________

Pre-Exercise Meal / Snack:_____________________

Energy Level Before Workout: L   M   H

Weight:________   Sleep:________   Calories:_______

Cardio

Type:______________________________________

Time:____________   Distance:_____________

Heart Rate:______________   Intensity: L   M   H

Strength Training

Exercise	Sets	Reps	Wt	Rest

Notes / Comments

____

____

____

Daily Workout Log

Date: _____________

Pre-Exercise Meal / Snack: _____________________________

Energy Level Before Workout: L   M   H

Weight: __________   Sleep: __________   Calories: __________

Cardio

Type: ____

Time: _______________   Distance: _______________

Heart Rate: _______________   Intensity: L   M   H

Strength Training

Exercise	Sets	Reps	Wt	Rest

Notes / Comments

____

____

____

Daily Workout Log   Date: ___________

Pre-Exercise Meal / Snack: ____________________________

Energy Level Before Workout: L   M   H

Weight: _________   Sleep: _________   Calories: ________

Cardio

Type: ____

Time: ______________   Distance: ______________

Heart Rate: ______________   Intensity: L   M   H

Strength Training

Exercise	Sets	Reps	Wt	Rest

Notes / Comments

____

____

____

Daily Workout Log

Date: _____________

Pre-Exercise Meal / Snack: _____________________________

Energy Level Before Workout: L   M   H

Weight: _________   Sleep: _________   Calories: _________

Cardio

Type: ____

Time: _______________   Distance: _______________

Heart Rate: _______________   Intensity: L   M   H

Strength Training

Exercise	Sets	Reps	Wt	Rest

Notes / Comments

____

____

____

Daily Workout Log　　Date: _________

Pre-Exercise Meal / Snack: ____________________

Energy Level Before Workout:　L　　M　　H

Weight: _______　　Sleep: _______　　Calories: _______

Cardio

Type: _______________________________

Time: ___________　　　　Distance: ____________

Heart Rate: ____________　　Intensity: L　　M　　H

Strength Training

Exercise	Sets	Reps	Wt	Rest

Notes / Comments

____

____

____

Daily Workout Log   Date: _________

Pre-Exercise Meal / Snack: _____________________

Energy Level Before Workout: L   M   H

Weight: _______   **Sleep:** _______   **Calories:** _______

Cardio

Type: _____________________________________

Time: ___________   **Distance:** ____________

Heart Rate: ___________   **Intensity:** L   M   H

Strength Training

Exercise	Sets	Reps	Wt	Rest

Notes / Comments

____

____

____

Daily Workout Log   Date: __________

Pre-Exercise Meal / Snack: ____________________

Energy Level Before Workout: L   M   H

Weight: ________   Sleep: ________   Calories: _______

Cardio

Type: ____

Time: ____________   Distance: ____________

Heart Rate: ____________   Intensity: L   M   H

Strength Training

Exercise	Sets	Reps	Wt	Rest

Notes / Comments

____

____

____

Daily Workout Log   Date: _________

Pre-Exercise Meal / Snack: _____________________

Energy Level Before Workout: L   M   H

Weight: _______   Sleep: _______   Calories: _______

Cardio

Type: _____________________________________

Time: ____________   Distance: ______________

Heart Rate: _____________   Intensity: L   M   H

Strength Training

Exercise	Sets	Reps	Wt	Rest

Notes / Comments

____

____

____

Daily Workout Log   Date: _____________

Pre-Exercise Meal / Snack: _____________________________

Energy Level Before Workout: L   M   H

Weight: _________   Sleep: _________   Calories: _________

Cardio

Type: ____

Time: _______________   Distance: _______________

Heart Rate: _______________   Intensity: L   M   H

Strength Training

Exercise	Sets	Reps	Wt	Rest

Notes / Comments

____

____

____

Daily Workout Log

Date: _____________

Pre-Exercise Meal / Snack: ______________________

Energy Level Before Workout: L   M   H

Weight: _________   Sleep: _________   Calories: _________

Cardio

Type: ______________________________________

Time: ______________   Distance: ______________

Heart Rate: ______________   Intensity: L   M   H

Strength Training

Exercise	Sets	Reps	Wt	Rest

Notes / Comments

____

____

____

Daily Workout Log   Date: __________

Pre-Exercise Meal / Snack: ____________________

Energy Level Before Workout: L   M   H

Weight: ________   Sleep: ________   Calories: ________

Cardio

Type: ____________________________________

Time: ____________   Distance: ____________

Heart Rate: ____________   Intensity: L   M   H

Strength Training

Exercise	Sets	Reps	Wt	Rest

Notes / Comments

____

____

____

Daily Workout Log   Date:______________

Pre-Exercise Meal / Snack:________________________

Energy Level Before Workout: L   M   H

Weight:__________   Sleep:__________   Calories:__________

Cardio

Type:____

Time:______________   Distance:________________

Heart Rate:__________________   Intensity: L   M   H

Strength Training

Exercise	Sets	Reps	Wt	Rest

Notes / Comments

____

____

____

Daily Workout Log

Date: _____________

Pre-Exercise Meal / Snack: _______________________

Energy Level Before Workout: L   M   H

Weight: _________   Sleep: _________   Calories: _________

Cardio

Type: ____

Time: _______________   Distance: _______________

Heart Rate: _______________   Intensity: L   M   H

Strength Training

Exercise	Sets	Reps	Wt	Rest

Notes / Comments

____

____

____

Daily Workout Log

Date: _____________

Pre-Exercise Meal / Snack: _____________________________

Energy Level Before Workout: L   M   H

Weight: _________   Sleep: _________   Calories: _________

Cardio

Type: ____

Time: _______________   Distance: _______________

Heart Rate: _______________   Intensity: L   M   H

Strength Training

Exercise	Sets	Reps	Wt	Rest

Notes / Comments

____

____

____

Daily Workout Log   Date: ___________

Pre-Exercise Meal / Snack: ________________________

Energy Level Before Workout: L   M   H

Weight: _________   Sleep: _________   Calories: _________

Cardio

Type: ____

Time: _____________   Distance: _______________

Heart Rate: _______________   Intensity: L   M   H

Strength Training

Exercise	Sets	Reps	Wt	Rest

Notes / Comments

____

____

____

Daily Workout Log

Date:______________

Pre-Exercise Meal / Snack:______________________

Energy Level Before Workout: L   M   H

Weight:_________   Sleep:__________   Calories:_________

Cardio

Type:____

Time:______________   Distance:______________

Heart Rate:________________   Intensity: L   M   H

Strength Training

Exercise	Sets	Reps	Wt	Rest

Notes / Comments

____

____

____

Daily Workout Log   Date: _____________

Pre-Exercise Meal / Snack: _____________________________

Energy Level Before Workout: L   M   H

Weight: _________   Sleep: _________   Calories: _________

Cardio

Type: ____

Time: _____________   Distance: _______________

Heart Rate: _______________   Intensity: L   M   H

Strength Training

Exercise	Sets	Reps	Wt	Rest

Notes / Comments

____

____

____

Daily Workout Log   Date: __________

Pre-Exercise Meal / Snack: ______________________

Energy Level Before Workout: L   M   H

Weight: ________   Sleep: ________   Calories: ________

Cardio

Type: ____

Time: ____________   Distance: ______________

Heart Rate: ______________   Intensity: L   M   H

Strength Training

Exercise	Sets	Reps	Wt	Rest

Notes / Comments

____

____

____

Daily Workout Log   Date: __________

Pre-Exercise Meal / Snack: ___________________________

Energy Level Before Workout: L   M   H

Weight: ________   **Sleep:** ________   **Calories:** ________

Cardio

Type: ____

Time: ___________   **Distance:** _____________

Heart Rate: ______________   **Intensity:** L   M   H

Strength Training

Exercise	Sets	Reps	Wt	Rest

Notes / Comments

____

____

____

Daily Workout Log

Date: _____________

Pre-Exercise Meal / Snack: _______________________

Energy Level Before Workout: L   M   H

Weight: _________   Sleep: _________   Calories: _________

Cardio

Type: _______________________________________

Time: _____________   Distance: _______________

Heart Rate: _______________   Intensity: L   M   H

Strength Training

Exercise	Sets	Reps	Wt	Rest

Notes / Comments

____

____

____

Daily Workout Log

Date: _____________

Pre-Exercise Meal / Snack: _____________________

Energy Level Before Workout: L   M   H

Weight: ________   Sleep: _________   Calories: ________

Cardio

Type: _______________________________________

Time: ______________   Distance: _______________

Heart Rate: _______________   Intensity: L   M   H

Strength Training

Exercise	Sets	Reps	Wt	Rest

Notes / Comments

____

____

____

Daily Workout Log

Date: _____________

Pre-Exercise Meal / Snack: _______________________

Energy Level Before Workout: L   M   H

Weight: _________   Sleep: _________   Calories: _________

Cardio

Type: ___________________________________

Time: _____________   Distance: _______________

Heart Rate: _______________   Intensity: L   M   H

Strength Training

Exercise	Sets	Reps	Wt	Rest

Notes / Comments

____

____

____

Daily Workout Log

Date: __________

Pre-Exercise Meal / Snack: __________________________

Energy Level Before Workout: L   M   H

Weight: ________   Sleep: ________   Calories: ________

Cardio

Type: ____

Time: ____________   Distance: ______________

Heart Rate: ______________   Intensity: L   M   H

Strength Training

Exercise	Sets	Reps	Wt	Rest

Notes / Comments

____

____

____

Daily Workout Log   Date: __________

Pre-Exercise Meal / Snack: ____________________

Energy Level Before Workout: L   M   H

Weight: ________   Sleep: ________   Calories: ________

Cardio

Type: ____________________________________

Time: ____________   Distance: ______________

Heart Rate: ______________   Intensity: L   M   H

Strength Training

Exercise	Sets	Reps	Wt	Rest

Notes / Comments

____

____

____

Day 60 Notes On Fitness Progress

Action Plan

Daily Workout Log

Date: _______________

Pre-Exercise Meal / Snack: _______________________

Energy Level Before Workout: L   M   H

Weight: _________   Sleep: _________   Calories: _________

Cardio

Type: ____

Time: _______________   Distance: _______________

Heart Rate: _______________   Intensity: L   M   H

Strength Training

Exercise	Sets	Reps	Wt	Rest

Notes / Comments

____

____

____

Daily Workout Log

Date: _____________

Pre-Exercise Meal / Snack: _____________________

Energy Level Before Workout: L   M   H

Weight: _________   Sleep: _________   Calories: _________

Cardio

Type: _________________________________

Time: _____________   Distance: _____________

Heart Rate: _______________   Intensity: L   M   H

Strength Training

Exercise	Sets	Reps	Wt	Rest

Notes / Comments

____

____

____

Daily Workout Log   Date: _____________

Pre-Exercise Meal / Snack: _______________________

Energy Level Before Workout: L   M   H

Weight: _________   Sleep: _________   Calories: _________

Cardio

Type: ____

Time: _____________   Distance: _______________

Heart Rate: _______________   Intensity: L   M   H

Strength Training

Exercise	Sets	Reps	Wt	Rest

Notes / Comments

____

____

____

Daily Workout Log   Date: _________

Pre-Exercise Meal / Snack: ____________________

Energy Level Before Workout: L   M   H

Weight: ________   Sleep: ________   Calories: ________

Cardio

Type: ______________________________________

Time: ____________   Distance: ______________

Heart Rate: ______________   Intensity: L   M   H

Strength Training

Exercise	Sets	Reps	Wt	Rest

Notes / Comments

____

____

____

Daily Workout Log   Date:___________

Pre-Exercise Meal / Snack: _______________________

Energy Level Before Workout: L   M   H

Weight:_________   Sleep:_________   Calories:_________

Cardio

Type:____

Time:_____________   Distance:________________

Heart Rate:________________   Intensity: L   M   H

Strength Training

Exercise	Sets	Reps	Wt	Rest

Notes / Comments

____

____

____

Daily Workout Log   Date: _____________

Pre-Exercise Meal / Snack: _______________________

Energy Level Before Workout: L   M   H

Weight: _________   Sleep: _________   Calories: _________

Cardio

Type: ____

Time: _______________   Distance: _______________

Heart Rate: _______________   Intensity: L   M   H

Strength Training

Exercise	Sets	Reps	Wt	Rest

Notes / Comments

____

____

____

Daily Workout Log

Date: _____________

Pre-Exercise Meal / Snack: _____________________

Energy Level Before Workout: L   M   H

Weight: _________   Sleep: _________   Calories: _________

Cardio

Type: _______________________________________

Time: _____________   Distance: _______________

Heart Rate: _______________   Intensity: L   M   H

Strength Training

Exercise	Sets	Reps	Wt	Rest

Notes / Comments

____

____

____

Daily Workout Log

Date: _____________

Pre-Exercise Meal / Snack: _____________________________

Energy Level Before Workout: L   M   H

Weight: _________   Sleep: _________   Calories: _________

Cardio

Type: ____

Time: _______________   Distance: _______________

Heart Rate: _______________   Intensity: L   M   H

Strength Training

Exercise	Sets	Reps	Wt	Rest

Notes / Comments

____

____

____

Daily Workout Log   Date: __________

Pre-Exercise Meal / Snack: ___________________

Energy Level Before Workout: L   M   H

Weight: _________   Sleep: _________   Calories: _________

Cardio

Type: _______________________________________

Time: _____________   Distance: _______________

Heart Rate: _______________   Intensity: L   M   H

Strength Training

Exercise	Sets	Reps	Wt	Rest

Notes / Comments

____

____

____

Daily Workout Log   Date: __________

Pre-Exercise Meal / Snack: ___________________

Energy Level Before Workout: L   M   H

Weight: ________   Sleep: ________   Calories: ________

Cardio

Type: _______________________________________

Time: ____________   Distance: _____________

Heart Rate: ______________   Intensity: L   M   H

Strength Training

Exercise	Sets	Reps	Wt	Rest

Notes / Comments

____

____

____

Daily Workout Log   Date: __________

Pre-Exercise Meal / Snack: ____________________

Energy Level Before Workout: L   M   H

Weight: ________   Sleep: ________   Calories: ________

Cardio

Type: ____

Time: ____________   Distance: ______________

Heart Rate: ______________   Intensity: L   M   H

Strength Training

Exercise	Sets	Reps	Wt	Rest

Notes / Comments

____

____

____

Daily Workout Log

Date: _____________

Pre-Exercise Meal / Snack: _____________________________

Energy Level Before Workout: L   M   H

Weight: _________   Sleep: _________   Calories: _________

Cardio

Type: ____

Time: _____________   Distance: _______________

Heart Rate: _______________   Intensity: L   M   H

Strength Training

Exercise	Sets	Reps	Wt	Rest

Notes / Comments

____

____

____

Daily Workout Log   Date: _____________

Pre-Exercise Meal / Snack: _______________________

Energy Level Before Workout: L   M   H

Weight: _________   Sleep: _________   Calories: _________

Cardio

Type: _______________________________________

Time: _______________   Distance: _______________

Heart Rate: _______________   Intensity: L   M   H

Strength Training

Exercise	Sets	Reps	Wt	Rest

Notes / Comments

____

____

____

Daily Workout Log   Date: __________

Pre-Exercise Meal / Snack: ____________________

Energy Level Before Workout: L   M   H

Weight: ________   Sleep: ________   Calories: ________

Cardio

Type: _______________________________________

Time: ____________   Distance: ______________

Heart Rate: ______________   Intensity: L   M   H

Strength Training

Exercise	Sets	Reps	Wt	Rest

Notes / Comments

____

____

____

Daily Workout Log

Date: __________

Pre-Exercise Meal / Snack: __________________________

Energy Level Before Workout: L   M   H

Weight: _________   Sleep: _________   Calories: _________

Cardio

Type: ____

Time: ______________   Distance: ______________

Heart Rate: ______________   Intensity: L   M   H

Strength Training

Exercise	Sets	Reps	Wt	Rest

Notes / Comments

____

____

____

Daily Workout Log   Date: _________

Pre-Exercise Meal / Snack: _____________________

Energy Level Before Workout: L   M   H

Weight: ________   Sleep: ________   Calories: _______

Cardio

Type: _______________________________________

Time: ____________   Distance: _____________

Heart Rate: ______________   Intensity: L   M   H

Strength Training

Exercise	Sets	Reps	Wt	Rest

Notes / Comments

____

____

____

Daily Workout Log

Date: ___________

Pre-Exercise Meal / Snack: ___________________________

Energy Level Before Workout: L   M   H

Weight: _________   Sleep: _________   Calories: _________

Cardio

Type: ____

Time: ______________   Distance: _______________

Heart Rate: _______________   Intensity: L   M   H

Strength Training

Exercise	Sets	Reps	Wt	Rest

Notes / Comments

____

____

____

Daily Workout Log   Date: _________

Pre-Exercise Meal / Snack: _______________________

Energy Level Before Workout: L   M   H

Weight: _________   Sleep: _________   Calories: _______

Cardio

Type: ____

Time: ____________   Distance: ____________

Heart Rate: ______________   Intensity: L   M   H

Strength Training

Exercise	Sets	Reps	Wt	Rest

Notes / Comments

____

____

____

Daily Workout Log   Date: __________

Pre-Exercise Meal / Snack: __________________________

Energy Level Before Workout: L   M   H

Weight: ________   Sleep: ________   Calories: ________

Cardio

Type: ____

Time: ____________   Distance: ______________

Heart Rate: ______________   Intensity: L   M   H

Strength Training

Exercise	Sets	Reps	Wt	Rest

Notes / Comments

____

____

____

Daily Workout Log   Date: __________

Pre-Exercise Meal / Snack: __________________________

Energy Level Before Workout: L   M   H

Weight: ________   Sleep: ________   Calories: ________

Cardio

Type: ____

Time: ____________   Distance: _______________

Heart Rate: _______________   Intensity: L   M   H

Strength Training

Exercise	Sets	Reps	Wt	Rest

Notes / Comments

____

____

____

Daily Workout Log　　　　Date: _________

Pre-Exercise Meal / Snack: _______________________

Energy Level Before Workout:　L　　M　　H

Weight: ________　Sleep: _________　Calories: ________

Cardio

Type: ____

Time: ____________　　　Distance: _____________

Heart Rate: _____________　Intensity: L　　M　　H

Strength Training

Exercise	Sets	Reps	Wt	Rest

Notes / Comments

____

____

____

Daily Workout Log   Date: _____________

Pre-Exercise Meal / Snack: _______________________

Energy Level Before Workout: L   M   H

Weight: _________   Sleep: _________   Calories: _________

Cardio

Type: ____

Time: _______________   Distance: _______________

Heart Rate: _______________   Intensity: L   M   H

Strength Training

Exercise	Sets	Reps	Wt	Rest

Notes / Comments

____

____

____

Daily Workout Log   Date: _________

Pre-Exercise Meal / Snack: ___________________

Energy Level Before Workout: L   M   H

Weight: _______   Sleep: ________   Calories: _______

Cardio

Type: ____

Time: ____________   Distance: _____________

Heart Rate: _______________   Intensity: L   M   H

Strength Training

Exercise	Sets	Reps	Wt	Rest

Notes / Comments

____

____

____

Daily Workout Log   Date: _________

Pre-Exercise Meal / Snack: ____________________

Energy Level Before Workout: L   M   H

Weight: _______   Sleep: _______   Calories: _______

Cardio

Type: ____________________________________

Time: ____________   Distance: ____________

Heart Rate: ____________   Intensity: L   M   H

Strength Training

Exercise	Sets	Reps	Wt	Rest

Notes / Comments

____

____

____

Daily Workout Log   Date:_______________

Pre-Exercise Meal / Snack:_________________________

Energy Level Before Workout: L   M   H

Weight:__________   Sleep:__________   Calories:__________

Cardio

Type:____

Time:________________   Distance:________________

Heart Rate:________________   Intensity: L   M   H

Strength Training

Exercise	Sets	Reps	Wt	Rest

Notes / Comments

____

____

____

Daily Workout Log   Date:_________

Pre-Exercise Meal / Snack:_________________________

Energy Level Before Workout: L   M   H

Weight:_______   Sleep:________   Calories:_______

Cardio

Type:____

Time:____________   Distance:______________

Heart Rate:______________   Intensity: L   M   H

Strength Training

Exercise	Sets	Reps	Wt	Rest

Notes / Comments

____

____

____

Daily Workout Log   Date:___________

Pre-Exercise Meal / Snack:_____________________________

Energy Level Before Workout: L   M   H

Weight:_________   Sleep:__________   Calories:_________

Cardio

Type:____

Time:_______________   Distance:________________

Heart Rate:________________   Intensity: L   M   H

Strength Training

Exercise	Sets	Reps	Wt	Rest

Notes / Comments

____

____

____

Daily Workout Log   Date: __________

Pre-Exercise Meal / Snack: _____________________

Energy Level Before Workout: L   M   H

Weight: ________   Sleep: ________   Calories: ________

Cardio

Type: ____

Time: ____________   Distance: ______________

Heart Rate: ______________   Intensity: L   M   H

Strength Training

Exercise	Sets	Reps	Wt	Rest

Notes / Comments

____

____

____

Daily Workout Log

Date: _____________

Pre-Exercise Meal / Snack: ___________________________

Energy Level Before Workout: L   M   H

Weight: _________   Sleep: _________   Calories: _________

Cardio

Type: ____

Time: _____________   Distance: _______________

Heart Rate: _______________   Intensity: L   M   H

Strength Training

Exercise	Sets	Reps	Wt	Rest

Notes / Comments

____

____

____

Daily Workout Log

Date: _____________

Pre-Exercise Meal / Snack: _______________________

Energy Level Before Workout: L   M   H

Weight: _________   Sleep: _________   Calories: _________

Cardio

Type: ____

Time: _______________   Distance: _______________

Heart Rate: _______________   Intensity: L   M   H

Strength Training

Exercise	Sets	Reps	Wt	Rest

Notes / Comments

____

____

____

Day 90 Notes On Fitness Progress

Action Plan

Notes

Notes

Notes

Notes

Notes

9 781709 994927